I0408422

Your Skin is Your Best Friend!

A Holistic Approach to Maintaining That Youthful Glow That We All Want & Love!

By Tonisha L. Dawson

Copyright © 2017 by Tonisha L. Dawson

Your Skin is Your Best Friend!

Copyright © 2017 by Tonisha L. Dawson

ISBN- 13: 978-1544914695

ISBN- 10: 1544914695

osunallureacademy.com

osunallurebeauty@gmail.com

Disclaimer: The author of this book has put together for informational and holistic purposed only. The author makes no guarantees or promises of results and will not be held liable for loss or damages. This work does not represent the expert opinion of a Physician or Dermatologist but the expert opinion of a Aesthetician and Holistic Life Coach and if the reader is in need of the former expert help, the author encourages the reader to seek a Physician or Dermatologist for services needed.

Your Skin is Your Best Friend!

Table of Contents

Your Skin is Your Best Friend!

Introduction

For thousands of years, the skin and its care has been a phenomenon especially as it relates to women. In Ancient times past skin care, eyebrow placement, hair color, cheek color, and lip color were all relative to your status in society and as it may seem not much has changed in society today as we are in the 20th Century.

There are literally thousands of products on the market all promoting something different as it relates to skin care and beauty, and most of them lure women in to spend hundreds of dollars yearly to maintain or create the illusion of the "perfect" looking skin and to reverse the signs of aging.

Let's be honest, some of these products work, and some of them don't, but we are willing to take the risk of trial and error until we found

Your Skin is Your Best Friend!

what works for us as it relates to our desired results.

This ultimately shows us how important beauty and our skin care are in general as it comes to our image and our everyday lives.

So let me ask you a question? How important is your skin care to you?

What are you willing to do to keep your skin looking its best for years to come?

It is one thing to buy makeup and foundation to even our skin tone and texture and to play with colors but it is another to actually have beautiful skin underneath all of that.

This book will unlock the inner and ancient secrets and techniques that will keep our skin in its most healthy and balanced state, and healthy skin is BEAUTIFUL skin! Healthy skin is vibrant, glowing, tight and YOUTHFUL skin!

Your Skin is Your Best Friend!

Isn't this our ultimate goal? Isn't this what we spend hundreds of dollars on yearly to look and feel our absolute best?

What if I told you there were natural alternatives that you can implement along with a favorite product that will give you fast and consistent results? Would you be willing to try them?

If so, let's delve into this exclusive skin care special report to get you the results that have been long awaited for!

Chapter 1

The Skin is a What!

As I stated in the introduction, skin care is a phenomenon that has been going on for literally thousands of years. Women in ancient times found the use of herbs, salves and tinctures to be particularly useful in maintaining and creating the most beautiful of skin. Our skin changes and actually has a mind of its own. It adapts to your environment, circumstances and surroundings and you surely have the ability to change the makeup of your skin in less than three months if you are consistent in its care!

Before I can go further about taking care of the skin, essentially, I have to educate you a little bit about your skin. Don't worry this will not be a lengthy synopsis of anatomy class but there are

Your Skin is Your Best Friend!

some basic principles and facts that you will NEED to know before moving forward.

Basically, the skin has four layers, the one that *we* deal with the most is the very top layer, although the other layers are extremely important as well. We do not physically touch these other layers and they are most affected by what we do from the *inside* out.

The very top layer of skin is what endures the most abuse because it is the layer that is exposed to the most.

Your skin is an organ, living moving and breathing. Most do not realize that the skin is an organ, although, it is the largest, spreading at about 20 feet if laid flat and performs numerous functions for the body itself. In short, the skin is super important. It keeps the insides in and the outside out. It is weather proof but is still able to be permeated. It is subject to many, many things and most of them can be harmful even if it is only down the line. It is subject to heat, cold, harsh conditions, chemicals, free radicals, germs, dirt, bacteria, pollution and a host of other things.

The skin is a tell all book about what is going on with you emotionally, physically and it surely tells a huge story about our overall health in general. The skin on your face being in the front line of the war, usually tells the most accurate story of how well you have cared for yourself with the rest of your skin to follow suit. Unless you have taken drastic measures such as pounds of makeup, dermatology treatments or cosmetic surgery treatments, your skin will not hide the disregard that you have for it by consuming chemicals, smoking, harsh sunlight, excessive drinking or just sheer neglect. Our skin works hard daily throughout our entire lifetime to be an effective defense to what it is exposed to regularly, it is our protective armor in this harsh environment that we live in. Our skin is a literal miracle worker that replenishes and renews **constantly** for our protection.

The skin that we live in is here for the long haul. Most of us will live long lengthy lives and our skin is required take that journey with us, wouldn't it be wonderful and make sense for us to keep it as healthy as possible while it hangs along for the ride?

Our skin when exposed to certain factors will change its makeup to suit that environment whether good or bad. The skin is always and constantly changing and it adapts to the needs of the person wearing it. This organ is indeed quite amazing! It is only when we begin to take our skin for granted that we will run into problems. Think about this, from the time we are born our skin is in its most perfect form at birth. It is new, supple, soft and does everything it is supposed to do unless of course there is a pre-existing condition, but even those comes from the actions of our parents before we were conceived. The skin from day one is attacked by elements, grows tougher and adapts from that moment forward. It is our job to give it the best care that we can so that is does not begin to deteriorate prematurely.

Let me ask you a question...Have you ever run into someone you went to high school with (which says that you are pretty close to the same age) and they look at least 10 years older? Or even worse yet, you may be on the opposite end of this scenario and see someone that YOU look 10 years older than, and you think to yourself, "what could they possibly be doing to keep their skin so youthful? This happens ALL of the time and the skin has shown and proven that the two of you have two totally different habits and lifestyles... unfortunately your skin had to defend itself accordingly.

Let's take a minute to discuss the functions of skin. The skin has many, the first of about six is Protection. The skin protects us from invasion of harmful bacteria, viruses, germs, UV radiation, etc. The second is Sensation. It allows us to feel... pressure, touch, heat, cold and pain. The third function is Temperature Regulation, this allows our body to retain or release heat depending on outside body temperature. The fourth is Immunity, the skin destroys microorganisms and interaction of the skin with the body's immune system. The fifth function is excretion, the skin excretes water, urea, ammonia and uric acid and the last function is absorption, absorption is limited but it does occur. Only certain substance can enter the body through the skin and influence the body to a minor degree. So now that we have the technical stuff out of the way, let's get into the fluffy stuff.

The skin is a phenomenon that we may never quite truly understand, however, it is *still* an organ and it is most definitely in our best interest to take care of our skin to the best of our ability.

It is not wise to consume alcoholic beverages regularly, permit extended exposure to the sun, smoking, extreme weather conditions or simply neglect. Our skin suffers greatly when we neglect to care for it.

Have you ever bought a new pair of Uggs, leather or suede shoes or boots? What is the first thing we do before we wear them if we care about keeping them for a while and getting good use out of them? We TREAT them! We put something on them to protect them from the weather conditions, damage or wear and tear. It is only fair to do at least the same for our skin! The sun as beautiful as it is and as wonderful as it is to go out on beach day, you owe it to yourself to wear sunscreen, put on a big brimmed hat, sit under an umbrella or anything else to protect the skin from the harmful rays of the sun. Extreme cold is no good either. It strips your skin of much needed moisture and can cause dry winter itch and pave the way for eczema or other scaly skin conditions. Skin during winter months should stay well hydrated and moisturized. This is a must! In any extreme weather conditions, you should protect your skin from the elements. This will prove to be beneficial to you in the long run.

The Makeup of Skin

Skin is comprised of four layers as well as layers within those layers. It is comprised of cells, keratin (which is a protein) and water. The way that skin works is, the innermost layer, I will not

name by its name because you will forget
anyway, creates new cells about every 28-30
days roughly. These new cells work their way up
to the outermost layer which will eventually
shed the old skin cells and replace them with the
new skin cells that were created. You follow me?
This is the cycle that goes on within our skin
about every month or so.

At the tender ages of birth to about 20-22, this
happens every single month like clockwork. We
are younger and our bodies more efficient, as we
age our bodies slow down and this process takes
slightly longer than a month.

This is where the aging process begins. Those
new cells take longer to produce and they take
their dear sweet time making it up to that outer
layer, because of this, the outer layer does not
shed off so quickly and you are left with older
skin cells that have been on your face longer,
because of this, the skin that has been making its

way to the top is not as new as well. This is how your skin's makeup begins to change, and this is when your skin begins to age.

Normal wear and tear of the skin starts to expose itself because the new cells are not being created as promptly. This is where you will begin to see dull, sagging skin. You may start to notice wrinkles or under eye circles, smile lines, crow's feet (wrinkles around the eyes) or your skin may lack luster in general.

This Is where the work on your end begins. Ultimately you will have to offer your skin some much needed assistance if you want to reverse what the body has slowed down naturally.

This slowing down process, again, starts at about the age of 20-22 and continues onward. Dedication needs to be put forth in order to keep this process moving at a successful rate and to reverse the signs of aging. Another very important fact, it is much easier to significantly slow down the aging process, than it is to reverse the signs of aging. Just food for thought.

Let me explain to you something... This information is going to be very important moving forward, this information will be the catalyst to change your skin and the founding reason for everything that I instruct you to do moving forward. This is one of the most important keys that you will need to know in order to transform your skin. Are you ready for this information?

Here goes: The skin creates new cells every 28-30 days as I stated earlier. What this means for us, is that we have new skin every 30 days. Stay with me. These skin cells that we have and produce are *replicated.* What this means is, every 30 days we have a completely new face! The reason that we don't see anything different is because our skin keeps replicating the same cells, the same skin, and ultimately the same face. The only way that you can trick and inevitably CHANGE the makeup and look of your skin is to develop a regime that works for your skin and keep up with it so that your skin will recreate the new cellular structure and continue to replicate those. This is not a hoax! This is anatomy, this is science! Let's talk about what needs to be done in order to facilitate this process.

Chapter 2

Skin Care is a Commitment

Let's talk about what it is going to take to have this beautiful skin that we all want and love.

Most women no matter what age, deal with some form of issues as it relates to their skin. These issues range from acne, large pores, under skin congestion, sensitivities, rosacea, hyperpigmentation, dryness, oiliness, and the list can go on. One or more of these issues plague most women at some point or another. It is very rare to find a woman or anyone for that matter that has the "perfect" skin. The skin is indeed a mystery. It changes based on climate and external factors, as well stress and diet. If one or more of these factors change, your skin may change as well.

21

Your Skin is Your Best Friend!

This is why taking proper care of your skin is of upmost importance. In order to keep up with the changes your skin makes on a daily, you have to be committed to this process.

Let's talk about the moment that you want to see change in your skin. You may have issues with hyperpigmentation (dark spots), occasional acne, large pores, under eye circles, small wrinkles or you may simply want a healthier glowing version of what you already have. You may also have skin issues in general on other parts of the body; dry, scaly, itchy skin, oily skin, sensitive skin, skin that is easily bruised, etc. When you want these things to change, there is a little bit of work that needs to be done on your part.

This work needs to be consistent and constant. You will NEVER see the results that you want if you are sporadic and inconsistent with your regimen. The regimen that you use will be different for everyone based on the results that you need, but I can assure you that whatever it is, it needs to be done on a consistent basis in order to see results.

Very often as I am working, I run into clients who want change in the skin especially as it relates to their face, I ask them one question… "What is your at home regimen?" The answer that I receive most often is "Oh, I don't do anything much at home" "I have products but I barely use them" Ummm……Ooookkkaaay. How do you expect to see results or any type of change in your skin if you don't do ANYTHING at home? This is almost always the next question in sequence. I love to help, and I WANT them to see results but if they will not help me help them, our entire process is in vain. I am not one to want to continue taking a client's money, knowing good and well that if they don't start to do something at home, all of my hard work will be null and void anyway. I can do my best to assist them in receiving results after my treatments, but there has to be some effort put in on their part as well. I cannot stress this enough!

The fact of the matter is, your skin is an everchanging organ and YOU have the power to assist in that change. It simply takes effort and dedication on your part.

It is understandable that in the hustle and bustle of life, children, careers, work schedules, school, extra-curricular activities and so on, we may not get the time to develop an extensive regimen or skin care routine, but you have to at least take about ten minutes aside each day to dedicate to your skin. I know that this may be a lot to ask because most of us barely even have the time to do the basics and necessities, but I beg you to start looking at this segment as a necessity as

Your Skin is Your Best Friend!

well. Your skin will surely thank you and reward you accordingly.

So, let's get right into this!

Your face needs to be cleansed daily, if you are on the oilier side, maybe even twice daily. Notice, that I did not say washed. Your face is not dirty and does not need a good washing. It needs to be balanced from the elements and things that occur to it from the outside. A good "cleanser" will do that for you. This part is important. It cleanses the skin, breaks up oil, sebum, dust and debris attracted to your skin over the course of the day. It clears the pores and refreshes the skin. It also helps with removing old skin cells and clearing out the pores. This should be done consistently...as consistently as possible. You do not want your skin replicating clogged pores, an unbalanced Ph or whatever your skin had to fight off for that

Your Skin is Your Best Friend!

day. It is best to cleanse the face daily and give it a fresh start and a fighting chance.

Secondly, the skin NEEDS to be exfoliated. This is the process of assisting the skin to shed the "older" skin cells that are supposed to slough off on their own. This is an imperative piece of the puzzle in anti-aging. It will also assist in keeping the skin young, fresh, glowing, and refined. Exfoliation should occur about once a week in the younger ages, and at least twice a week in the older ages. The way that this regimen works is by getting rid of the old skin cells that have not shed off on their own, once this occurs, the skin instantly goes to work creating "new" skin to replace that skin that was lost. Having a consistent exfoliation regime will "glow" your skin up in no time and have you looking younger and more vibrant than ever!

Our next step is a specialty step which may include, a mask, serum or peel.

Your Skin is Your Best Friend!

Let's be very clear, you DO NOT need ALL of these products in order to have an effective regimen, but it is nice to have at least one specialty product in your beauty cabinet. A mask is to be used about once a week and can be used to combat issues like oiliness, anti-aging, acneic skin, sensitive skin, large pores, skin tightening and many other things. They are a great go to product when you are away on vacation or can be used for simple spot treatments, they are an awesome product to have in your regimen.

Serums, are great because they are finely formulated and usually very, very potent and very, very expensive. The reason for this is because they usually use expensive, and potent products in the serum and the molecules are small enough to actually penetrate the skin at the dermal level to produce results. They are usually rich in antioxidants, essential oils, honeys and natural or aggressive products based on which line you use.

Peels, usually filled with some sort of natural acid either fruit based on synthetic to resurface the skin at a more deeper level than a regular exfoliant will. It resurfaces the skin slightly more assertive than the manual exfoliation of an exfoliant would. There is usually no manual manipulation with peels and they are left to sit on the face while acids or enzymes promote cell renewal. They are all very good and quite frankly are successful at getting the job done.

The last piece of your regimen is your moisturizer. The biggest misconception about moisturizer is that you do not need one if you have oily skin. This is not true, even if you have oily skin, you still need a moisturizer, simply one that is formulated for oily skin. There are usually specific ingredients that are in the formulation that will assist in combatting your oily skin. If your skin is indeed dry, this is definitely a product that you do not want to skip. After cleansing and exfoliating, your skin is depleted of much needed moisture and you need to replenish that moisture by using a moisturizer that is formulated for your particular skin type. This is super important.

These are your basic steps for at home maintenance, however I am in no way telling you that you have to implement all of these steps every night. The only imperative steps are cleansing and moisturizing, as well as one specialty step at least once a week. This should take a load off. Once a week adding a specialty and daily cleansing should not take its toll on you. This is the least you can do for something that is going to protect you and be around for as long as you are. Your skin needs this to be on its best behavior.

Your Skin is Your Best Friend!

The same goes for the skin on your body. It is affected by the clothing that we wear, the dyes in the clothing, the weather, laundry detergents and so on. It is of upmost importance to take care of your body as well. Your body needs to be bathed regularly, but it is also a major misconception that it has to be bathed every day. It is a matter of preference but not required. Water should not be scalding hot, although I am guilty of this myself, super hot water dries the skin out and depletes it of its natural moisture, so tread softly with this.

Skin after bathing should always be moisturized, preferably while the body is still damp. This will seal in the moisture that is lost during the bathing process. Lotions are good, but creams, body butter and oils work best as they are thicker and have more emollients. The emollients penetrate the skin as well as sit on top of the skin for extra moisturization. This will work wonders for your skin as you age. Be sure to thoroughly massage the cream into the skin, as massaging will help with circulation, combat cellulite and assist with tightening and firming the skin. By simply creaming your body you can assist in your overall health.

The skin will stay tighter, firmer and keep its tone by caring for it effectively. You will not have to worry about saggy, loose or flaccid skin that has lost its elasticity if you begin to give it that care it needs and deserves.

As a skin care specialist, I am obsessed with having healthy skin. Healthy skin is plump, full, firm and glowing skin. Many people, once they find out my daily regimen, openly admit that it is too much and do not have this type of dedication. I take a bath every night, not because I feel as though I need one, but I take it to relax and allow my skin the moisture that it needs. I usually add some form of oil to my bath either, coconut, olive, grapeseed, almond or jojoba. Usually whatever I have lying around works. Water and oil do not mix so this process allows the oil to sit on top of the skin and trap the moisture inside. I use my soap as usual, but I add the step of an in-shower lotion, this lotion goes on and rinses off. After I get out of the bath, I towel dry, still remaining damp and apply my moisturizer, following this, I add my body oil to top it all off. This allows the oil to remain on my skin so that I do not wake up dry and/or ashy in the morning. Most days I take a shower in the morning but not always. The days that I do take a morning shower, I add the in-shower body lotion again and I still moisturize although I forgo the oil. This allows my skin to have a constant residual of moisture and I barely experience dryness or skin issues.

This brings me to my next topic. Season Changes. When the seasons change, guess what? Your skin changes. In Fall our skin detoxes and regulates, Winter it is dries out, Spring our skin purges and Summer our skin flourishes and blossoms. Why is that? The first reason is climate changes, the second is diet changes which we will delve into more deeply in our next chapter.

Let's talk about climate change. Fall is a season where things get prepared for the winter season. Leaves brighten and fall off of the trees, animals prepare for hibernation and fruits and plants lose their seeds. The same goes for our skin. It begins to prepare itself for the winter months. It may produce more oil, balances itself, detoxes and gets ready for the dry winter months. In Winter, the skin is depleted. There is not much nourishment, and virtually no moisture. The air is colder and drier and sucks the life out of your skin. In Spring months, your skin has gone from extremely dry to warmer weather. The skin starts to produce more sebum, it may begin to sweat and breakout. In Summer the skin has begun to regulate, our diet changes and we drink more water. Our skin is hydrated and luscious in summer months.

 I will repeat, skin care is a commitment. Great skin does not occur merely by happenstance. There is time and dedication that has to be put forth to receive the results that you desire. Your skin can evolve into whatever you would like it to be, it just takes a little more effort on your part. Take some time to dedicate to the nurturing of your skin. Your skin will in turn reward you, Trust me!

Chapter 3

Healing Inside Out, the Holistic Approach

Our ever- changing skin needs our assistance in order to flourish to its highest potential. The most imperative thing that we can do to help in in this manner is to also heal it from the inside out. There has been an old-school adage if you will, that you are what you eat. There is much truth to this statement, as everything that we consume affects us in different ways.

The things that we eat and drink are, in essence, like watering a plant. The more good you put in the more good you get out, the more bad you put in the more bad that you get out. This simply means that what we decide to eat and drink can affect our skin positively or negatively.

Your Skin is Your Best Friend!

Think about it; in Summer months your skin glows and your hair grows. Why do you think this is? This is mainly because our diet usually changes significantly in Summer. We drink tons more water because of the heat, we eat lighter and healthier, various fruits and vegetables are more accessible to us and we receive and synthesize more Vitamin D from the Sun. When we eat healthier, we ARE healthier, it is as simple as that.

In Winter months, we eat heavier, drink less because of the cold and Vitamin D is virtually non-existent. Our bodies take longer digesting the food, causing important vitamins and nutrients to be delayed getting where they need to go. All of this in turn affects our skin.

I can always tell what is going on in a client's life based on the story that their skin tells me. I can tell if they are stressed, hormonal, or if they smoke, drink etc. The skin is like a tell all book of what you do to it at home.

Clients that smoke or drink on a regular or live in the house with someone that smokes in the home, their skin will lack luster and have no glow to it whatsoever. The reason for this is because when a person smokes or drinks excessively, the capillaries in the skin constrict, disallowing sufficient blood flow to those areas and the skin will lose its luster.

Clients are always baffled when I ask them if they drink or smoke during their facial or consultation. They are always curious as to how I am privy to this information. I have to explain to them that I know this information based on what their skin has revealed to me. Blackheads may be more prominent, and the blackheads will smell like cigarette smoke. The skin will not plump as much during manipulations, and it will not look as rejuvenated once the facial is complete. This is because the blood cannot flow as fast or as thoroughly as it can with normal skin. This is also, because skin is responsible for secretions and excretions, cigarette smokers excrete the toxins from the cigarette and nicotine onto their skin and also experience deeper skin issues with blackheads, papules, milia and inflamed areas.

Heavy drinkers experience the same issues with lackluster and dull skin cells. Excessive drinking slows down the sloughing off process and skin will not be a vibrant because of this.

Once again, our diet plays a very big part in our healing processes. All of our organs and functions are interconnected in a magical way and when one is not functioning correctly, they all suffer in one way or another, your skin being the largest, with the most functions is one of them.

Your Skin is Your Best Friend!

So, let's talk a little bit about this diet that I continue to mention. As it relates to what you eat, foods should be high in nutritional content for your skin to benefit the most. If you do not receive all that you need from the foods that you eat, a supplement may be in order. Vitamins are a good way to supplement nutritional deficiencies. Processed foods should be limited as well as sodas, junk food and fast foods. They usually have minimal nutritional content and are filled with things that your body struggles to process. Foods that are rich in Vitamin C, A, K, B and Iron are great to add to your diet, as well as leafy greens, fresh fruits and lean proteins.

Eating loads of fast food, sweet and carbonated beverages, as well as loads of sweets puts unnecessary strain on your other organs to process and digest them and in turn ends up affecting your skin. Once again, your skin tells a story and the foods that you eat will surely show on your face soon than later. It is all relative. Taking care of your skin from the inside out is what counts, and taking care of your skin from the outside in comes secondary. If you are consistent at both your skin will thank you and reward you as a result of.

What many people fail to realize is that the majority of skin issues are determined by things that you eat, even children with allergies, bad eczema, and scaly itchy skin is usually a result of an allergy of food that is consumed. Change your diet and you can change your skin.

The human body replaces cells every day all day, every day the body replaces over 3.5 billion cells, because of this every 30 days you have a new face, every 6 to 9 months you have new skin and organs and every 7 years you have an entire new body. If you make the dedication to start today from this day forward to do the right thing by your body, your skin, and your health in general, you can completely change anything about your body that is ailing you. This is great news to know! If you continue to stay diligent, and consistent in your work, you can change any ailment, sickness, disease, weight change, skin structure or anything else that you would like to see a difference in.

The next topic I would like to explore in greater detail is your supplements. As I stated earlier, if you are not receiving the proper nourishment from the food that you eat, you can supplement with vitamins. Let's talk about some vitamins and the benefits that they will have for you. (found on Google)

Vitamin A has many benefits. It assists with good vision, is essential for reproduction, has a role in cell growth and cell division, supports the immune system and supports health of the skin. It is also good for healthy bone growth. Vitamin A is the active ingredient used for Retinol which assist in treating acne and psoriasis. Top Vitamin A foods are Carrots, Kale, Spinach, Broccoli, Butter, Eggs, Sweet Potatoes and Squash.

Vitamin B usually taken as a complex, consist of eight B vitamins. B1 (thiamine), B2 (riboflavin), B3 (niacin), B5 (pantothenic acid), B6 , B7 (biotin), B9 (folate), B12 . Vitamin B keeps our bodies running and converts our food into fuel for us. There is usually a B deficiency in older adults, Vegans, Vegetarians, heart failure and alcoholism. Deficiencies are linked to depression, acne, anxiety, fatigue, heart disease, PMS and skin problems. The benefits include increased energy, improved memory, stimulates immune system and boost your hair and skin health. Foods rich in Vitamin B are beef liver, sardines, red meat, salmon, milk, soy, swiss cheese, and yogurt.

Vitamin C is necessary for the growth, repair, and development of all body tissues. it assists in many body functions, the absorption of iron, wound healing, the immune system, the formulation of collagen, and the maintenance of bones and teeth. A Vitamin C deficiency results in loss of collagen, easy bruising, bleeding gums, slow wound healing, dry hair, and nosebleeds. The benefits of consuming Vitamin C promote healthy glowing skin, and collagen formation, fights free radical damage, boost immunity, vital for circulation and heart health. Foods rich in Vitamin C are oranges, red peppers, kale, brussel sprouts, Broccoli, strawberries, grapefruit, guava, kiwi, and green peppers.

Vitamin D is important for the regulation of calcium and maintenance of healthy bones and teeth. It also provides protection from multiple diseases such as cancer, type 1 diabetes and multiple sclerosis. Deficiency symptoms include infections, skeletal diseases, metabolic disorders, cancer and cardiovascular disease. Foods rich in

Your Skin is Your Best Friend!

Vitamin D are fatty fish, cheese, egg yolk, salmon, sardines, tuna, mushrooms and sunlight.

Vitamin E is a fat soluble antioxidant which can only be obtained as a food supplement. The most widely known health benefits of vitamin e are protection against toxins, PMS, eye disorders such as cataracts, neurological diseases such as Alzheimer's disease and diabetes.

Biotin (B7) The benefit of Biotin is to thicken Hair, Nails and beautify the skin.

Evening Primrose Oil Women use evening primrose oil for PMS, breast pain, endometriosis, and symptoms of menopause such as hot flashes. It is an essential source of fatty acids, it is also used in soaps in cosmetics.

Black Cohash is most often used to control the symptoms of menopause such as headaches, hot flashes, mood changes, sleep problems, heart palpitations, nights sweats and vaginal dryness.

Your Skin is Your Best Friend!

The vitamins that I named above are just your most basic and there are many more supplements that can be taken to contribute to your overall health.

Don't waste any more time, start your lifestyle change today. Make a decision to eat a little more healthy and take supplements if you have to. Lay off the fast and processed foods and switch over to natural fruits and vegetables. Your body, your skin, and your overall health will thank you for it in the future.

Chapter 4

Natural Remedies

In my personal and professional opinion, natural is always best. I love whole food markets and health food stores because I know that the products will be as close to their purest form as possible. I am also a huge fan of do it yourself products that are efficient and highly effective. Think about it, there are tons of beauty products on the market and quite frankly it can be overwhelming when it comes down to choosing what may work for you personally. They all have gimmicks, some form of hype or claim of a miraculous result and it's no wonder it can be hard to choose! Eventually you will have tried hundreds of products only to have a beauty cabinet stocked full of products that you no longer use because they have failed to deliver in one way or another.

The most important thing to remember and the best advise that I can give you, is to choose what works best for you, whether a high-end product or a drugstore product they all have the capacity to be effective in one way or another. I also want you to remember that the most effective way to assist ANY product in working for you is to *manipulate* the skin. Manipulation of the skin will promote blood flow, improve circulation and firm and tone skin. Wherever there is great blood flow, there is healing, freshness, and overall health. Our bodies become a little more sluggish as we age and manipulation of the skin helps with putting a slight fire to that sluggishness, adding that fire to a product that *actually* works, will work nothing in short of a miracle for your skin.

Your Skin is Your Best Friend!

The best part about this entire ordeal is that, most products that will correspond to your skin, are easily accessible to you and possibly right in your very own kitchen!

You will be amazed at the potency and effectiveness of natural herbs, oils, fruits, and vegetables and because they are in their purest form, you will reap the benefits of the potency without the additions of additives and preservatives. I am going to give you the benefits of certain products as well as some products that you can make in your own timing and in your own space. The best part about this is, you can make them as needed without loads of products lying around collecting dust.

Let's delve into some essential products that will be super effective in your skin care routine.

- **Coconut Oil**- Coconut oil has tons of benefits and if coconut oil does not work for you, you are more than likely allergic or have an aversion to it. It has hundreds of benefits literally so it would be virtually impossible for me to tell you all of them in this read, however, it works wonders for your skin and hair. In short Coconut oil has unique fatty compositions that allow it to penetrate skin and hair. Coconut oil moisturizes skin and is a natural antioxidant making it great for stopping wrinkles and skin irritations. It can assist in speedy healing for Herpes 1 and 2 and if ingested can inhibit the growth of cancerous cells, help with immune support, digestive issues and contributes to focus as well as mental performance.

- **Olive Oil-** Olive Oil is packed with anti-aging antioxidants and hydrating squalene making t a superb product for skin and hair. Olive oil helps smooth hair, soften cuticles, remove makeup, intensely moisturizes skin as it helps to seal in moisture, calms irritated and inflamed skin (it is my oil of choice after a Brazilian wax), it also fights aging because of the large amounts of Vitamin E and polyphenols which helps fights free radicals that damages the skin and advance the signs of aging.

- **Grapeseed Oil-** Grapeseed Oil has been around for ages with many benefits. It is light and easily absorbable. It can be used for acne, to minimize under eye circles, skin tightening and toning, as well as anti-aging. Grapeseed oil grows hair faster, combats dandruff, imparts shine to hair, helps to strengthen hair and is a natural conditioner.

- **Sea Salt-** Sea Salt is great for skin conditions and a sea salt bath can help immensely relieve eczema, and psoriasis. It opens up the pores, improves circulation in the skin and hydrates the tissues so that your skin can heal.

- **Apple Cider Vinegar-** Apple Cider Vinegar has many uses in skin care. It will make your skin feel smoother, absorb excess oil and reduce fine lines and wrinkles. It restores the proper PH level to your skin helping to counter further skin damage. A spot treatment can be used for age spots, pimples or acne scars overnight.

- **Avocado-** Benefits of avocado include anti-aging. Avocado is an amazing treatment that helps reduce wrinkles. Not only you can apply mashed avocado flesh to your skin as a facial mask, but also, when you eat avocado, it will help fight aging process from within

- **Cucumbers-** What people don't know is that cucumbers are like 90% water. but also contains ascorbic acid (vitamin C) and caffeic acid, both of which help soothe skin irritations and reduce swelling–these acids prevent water retention, which may explain why cucumbers applied topically are often helpful for swollen eyes, burns and dermatitis.

- **Black Tea-** Black Tea, fights free radicals, rooibos clears up acne, and the caffeine it contains helps minimize puffiness.

- **Green Tea-** has anti-aging and antioxidant benefits that can help delay signs of skin aging, such as sagging skin, sun damage, age spots, fine lines and wrinkles. The polyphenols in green tea help neutralize harmful free radicals, which can cause significant damage to the skin and accelerate the aging process.

- **Coffee Grounds-** Old coffee grounds make an excellent facial exfoliant, gently slouching off dead skin cells to reveal the fresh, healthy looking skin underneath.

These are just a few key ingredients that you may have lying around in your very own kitchen that will prove to be very effective for your skin and hair. The most you will need is possibly a hand mixer and containers to store your products away. It is very important to label products that you create yourself, they have a strong capacity to go bad or rancid and the last thing that you would want to expose your face to is a foul smelling product that has gone bad because of lack of use. It is best to make a small amount and use it at one sitting, this way you can ensure that you are using a fresh product.

Exfoliants, scrubs and bath salts are easiest to make. If you have brown sugar, Epsom salt or sea salt and some oil lying around, you are in business! Add some essential oils to the mix and you have yourself a customized product to suit your individual and personalized needs.

- Exfoliants can be made with used coffee grounds, sugar, ground tea, and even salt. (although I wouldn't use salt as my go to because it may sting the eyes if entered accidentally) Add a little bit of water and few drops of essential oils and

Voila! You have made yourself a product that will assist with anti-aging and cause your skin to feel like butter afterwards.

Bath Salts Can be made very easily. Grab about a ½ pound of Sea Salt or Epsom Salt and a few drops of essential oils and sprinkle about a cup of these salts into your bath and allow the aroma and the healing power of the oils to transform your condition.

Body Scrubs Can be made using sea salt and or brown sugar. Pour salt or sugar or combination of both (salt tends to be coarser) into a container, add your oil of choice either Coconut, Grapeseed, Jojoba or Almond and essential oils. Cinnamon is a great additive to a body scrub as it brings oxygen and blood to the surface of the skin helping to plump it.

- **Face Masks-** Face masks can be really simple to make but may take a tad bit more effort. The best masks to try are things that are luxurious for the face as well as refining and tightening. Here are a few ingredients that will call for a wonderful facial mask treatment that can be made in your kitchen.

Hydrating Facial Mask- ½ Avocado, 1tsp Plain Organic Yogurt, 1tsp Honey (raw honey works best) mash the avocado until its soft and add the yogurt and honey and blend together until it forms a paste. Apply to face and leave on for 10-15 minutes if you would like an extra dose of hydration add 1 or 2 tsp of Extra Virgin Olive Oil which instantly softens and smooths skin.

Oily Skin Mask- Oatmeal, Lemon Juice and Honey Facial Mask For Oily Skin: This is a very effective oily skin face mask. Simply combine organic oatmeal, honey and lemon juice. Apply this mixture on your face, taking care around and on the eyes area. Let the mask sit on your face for 10 minutes, and then rinse it off with warm water.

Mask for Acne- 2Tbsp Honey (Raw is best) 2Tbsp Nutmeg, 2Tbsp Milk. Use this honey milk mask to fight off acne. Honey naturally kills off bacteria to prevent future breakouts and nutmeg acts a gentle exfoliator that works for sensitive skin. Let this mask sit on for about 10-15 minutes, rinse off and follow up with your favorite moisturizer.

Pore Tightening Mask- 1 Egg White, 1tsp Orange juice, ½ Tsp Tumeric Powder.

Egg white proteins work great on oily skin types because it tightens pores and zaps acne-causing bacteria, whisk it with orange juice and turmeric (an herb that has brightening properties and evens out skin tone) Leave on the skin for 10-15 minutes and rinse off. Try to wear an old t-shirt because the turmeric stains.

- Skin or Hair Moisturizer- Skin and hair moisturizers can literally be made in a flash in your kitchen. I absolutely love making DIY (DO it Yourself) products. They are simple and you know exactly what they contain.
  Shea Butter- Is a superfood that is naturally rich in Vitamins A, E and F. It provides UV protection and provides the skin with essential fatty acids. It also works wonders for skin conditions like

eczema or psoriasis with its anti-inflammatory properties. Inflammatory issues are the main symptoms of skin and scalp conditions and since shea butter has no added chemicals it also makes it ideal for sensitive skin.

It is very effective at healing and curing conditions that directly affect the skin and scalp such as

- Burns
- Dermatitis
- Dry Skin
- Eczema
- Insect Bites/Stings
- Scars and Sores
- Skin Allergies and Rashes
- Skin Cracks

Your Skin is Your Best Friend!

It is very soothing to the skin and provides the skin with the antioxidants and emollients that it needs.

It is very simple to make your own hair or skin moisturizer and it only takes the minimal of products to use and you can have the perfect creamy, rich, luxurious, delicious cream that will work wonders on your skin and hair.

8oz Shea Butter

4oz Coconut Oil

4oz Almond or Jojoba Oil

½ Cup Aloe Vera Juice or Gel

1tsp Argan Oil

Add Essential Oils to your liking

Put mixture into a big bowl and use a hand held mixer to blend products together until it reaches a rich creamy consistency.

These are ONLY a few of the things that you can do for yourself at home. Good skin care products are surely not far beyond our reach and the more you explore and understand what the benefits of these ingredients will do for you, you can mix and match and concoct as you please! Gone are the days where we have to spend thousands of dollars on products that we have no use for or are ineffective to us. There are many books, You Tube pages and blogs or websites dedicated to home remedies for your face and skin.

If you need a more assertive treatment, I implore you to seek out a skin care specialist or Aesthetician, someone who is trained in the art of skin care and treatments. They will no doubt give you advise on a regimen that will work for your personal skin type and your personal needs.

Your Skin is Your Best Friend!

I have given you much needed information in this book and it was short, sweet and to the point. My job is to get you started on the right track with taking care of your skin it the most basic way and working your way up to allowing skin care to become a priority in your life. Remember, the skin NEVER lies, and most problems that occur with our skin are a result of an inner issue that needs to be dealt with even if it's something as simple as drinking more water or quitting smoking. Your skin tells a story. What story is your skin telling about you?

Your Skin is Your Best Friend!

Tonisha Dawson

Holistic Life Coach/ Aesthetician and Master Beauty Specialist

Osunallurebeauty@gmail.com

Osunallureacademy.com